I Can
Make You
THIN
For Life

By

Danial Barron Howe

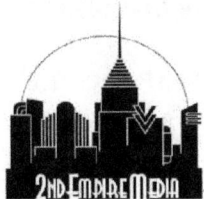

Important Notice!

The information and/or products outlined in this book is designed to be used in conjunction with, not instead of, your doctor's program. If you have an illness, then seek a doctor's care.

Do not use this information as a sole therapy against any disease or medical condition.

The information contained in this book is not recommended to diagnose, treat, cure or prevent any disease.

To purchase the full expanded 30 day program or the 90 Day Body program and receive free bonus software see our site at:

www.The30DayBurn.Com

About The Author

Danial Barron Howe is the author of over 350 books ranging from business to health and wellness. He is the founder of six multinational businesses including 2ndEmpireMedia, the publisher of this book.

Danial holds several degrees including a Masters in mechanical engineering and design as well as degrees in psychology and biomechanics. He is a lifelong tinkerer with a passion for improving efficiencies of systems such as those found here in this book.

INDEX

Results in just 7 days – Guaranteed!

Prepare yourself to read things you've likely NEVER read in a diet book before. I'm going to slay some sacred cows... and what the hell, we're even going to eat them and STILL manage to lose weight!

This little kindle book is my way of reaching out to people who buy book after book and program after program trying to discover some sort of "magic formula" for lifelong weight loss that seems to evade them year after year. – I have great news for you: *You just found it!*

Why I needed this information maybe even more that you!

A mere 6 months before creating *the 90 day body series* I underwent an intense look at my life, my lifestyle and the whole prospect of losing weight without expending any physical effort. It's not because I'm lazy mind you, I have a physical condition – degenerative bone disease. When I first started out, jogging, cardio and lifting weights was absolutely out of the question!

At 6 foot 10 inches tall (and originally tipping the scales at 305 pounds!) my joints are literally locked from full movement by calcium buildup as a byproduct of the condition that caused my extreme growth, making it impossible for me to do pushups or any type of real hardcore activity that's prescribed by literally all of the "diet experts". For me diet and diet ALONE would be the *only way* to save myself from a certain death by diet!

I'll tell you more about me here in a little bit. But right now let's talk about how I'm going to help you change your life.

I designed this simple 7 day "demo" to win you over and propel you to the next level.

I'm just like most people, I want quick results in everything I do. When it comes to weight loss my desires were really no different. I expect you're pretty much the same, so I've taken the best of what I've learned from my team of advisors and my own research and distilled it into this little book.

<u>My goals for you for the next 7 days are simple:</u>

- **Establish credibility with you by PROVING that what I say is true** - You'll see the changes happen *every single day* for the next 7 days. (It's hard to doubt what you witness with your own eyes!)
- **Get you to drop 7 to 10 pounds without lifting a finger** – Once you discover that cardio, weights, pills and workout equipment of all shapes and sizes are not the answer, your mind will begin to open to everything else I have to teach you.
- **I want your rave reviews!** That's right. I said it. I want you to shout it from the roof tops! And why wouldn't you? In 7 days you're going to discover how to *transform your body literally at will* - no matter how much you weigh or how much time you have in a day. (I lost most of my weight sitting in an office chair all day!)

Why 7 days?

Well, why not? It's only one week of your life. If you're *really serious* about finally doing something about that gut or those big thighs then you can hang in there for at least that long right? Sure you can!

But, here's the key to it all that I want you to keep in mind: *Take simple small steps*
If you follow along and do as I say then in 7 days you'll be looking at a new you – lighter by possibly 10 around pounds or more

If you continued on for 2 weeks that's 20 pounds off.
By week 3 that's 30 pounds.
By week 4 that would be a massive 40 pounds!
… and so on and so on…
That's how I did it; by concentrating ONLY on the next *mini goal* and NOT the total task.
As a famous televangelist used to say *"Inch by inch it's a cinch!"*

I recall each day checking my results on the scale and setting the next day's goal of shaving off another 1 to 2 pounds. Keeping clear each day of what my mission was went a long way to helping me maintain discipline and focus throughout the day as well.

As I sit here today I am 80 pounds lighter and still successfully moving toward my final 200 pound goal. I can say with absolute certainty that this method has made ALL the difference in the world!

Let me give you this one last bit of "pep talk" before we begin:

You're going to read things within these pages that may be new to you and no doubt you'll call them into question.

ALL I ASK YOU TO DO IS SUSPEND BELIEF AND JUST DO AS I ASK FOR NOW – THAT'S IT. NO BELIEF IS NEEDED UP FRONT. THAT PART WILL COME ON ITS OWN SOON ENOUGH.

Also, If you are thinking to yourself that you somehow fall into a "special" group of people and that this program couldn't possibly not produce results for you, then let me call your attention to the fact that WE ALL GOT FAT THE SAME WAY! … Right?

Every one of us are members of the same human family with the same basic biological make up. If the weight went on the same for me as it did for you, it will come off of you exactly the same way as it did for me and countless others…*period!*

Now let's get started. I can't wait to introduce you to a *thinner you* next week!

My Story

I'm sure you're just like me. For years you've looked at yourself in the mirror and you thought *"I really need to do something about this gut!"* Or maybe you even took it to the next level and actually bought some exercise equipment or a gym membership. But before long other things became more important and that new treadmill in the corner of your bedroom became an over glorified coat rack, or worse yet, it's been sitting in the basement collecting dust and cobwebs as you just invent excuse after excuse to not take action.

I'm going to share a secret with you (well, actually it's not really much of a secret at all) *exercising sucks!* It's time-consuming, it's painful, and let's be honest, there is at least a million other more pleasurable things you would rather be doing than grinding out 30 minutes on a treadmill just to drop half the amount of calories that you can find in a king-size snicker's bar – *which by the way takes less than three minutes to eat!* Hardly seems like a fair tradeoff does it? All that pain for just a few minutes of pleasure.

My Story

Like many of you I have battled my weight my entire life. I was a skinny kid up until the age of five when my parents bought a restaurant and we lived below it. I had unlimited access to far more food than any kid should possibly ever have and a mother that equated love with having well fed children. It proved to be a toxic combination.

Because I was a large child *(as an adult I now stand*

over 6'10!) my parents never questioned my voracious appetite. "He's a growing boy" they would say, "let him eat!" And so I did. This went on unchecked for years until in high school I found myself weighing 275 pounds, mostly fat. It was awkward enough to be over a foot taller than most kids, let alone bordering on morbidly obese as well.

It was the mid-1980s then and diet pills such as *Dexitrim* (the original stuff with Fen/Phen!) had hit the market and I was desperate to make a change. So I bought a box. I remember the instructions quite clearly; *"Take two pills in the morning and two in the afternoon. Maintain a diet of 1200 calories or less!"* So that's exactly what I did…

I recall sitting in class my junior year of high school - my heart pounding like a racehorse yet my eyes barely able to remain open from the extreme shock I was putting my body through by incorporating such a radical change in my diet. I had gone from 5 to 6 "meals" a day to less than one for the whole day! In my infinite wisdom I decided to start every day with a can of Diet Coke and a bag of peanut M&Ms and nothing else… I would skip lunch and then on the way home I'd have a single small McDonald's hamburger- no lettuce, no tomato, just meat and bun - *sans fries* as well on most days as well.

Later most evenings, if I could manage to hold my eyes open, I would attempt to do my homework and afterward collapse from exhaustion usually by 7 PM. This went on for well over 30 days. I was surviving on sheer willpower, *but it was working!* The weight was coming off and people were beginning to notice. More importantly, *Girls* were beginning to notice! This only fueled my resolve to continue the madness. In retrospect it was pure dietary suicide.

Something's got to give!

Around day 60 and some 90 pounds lighter, I made my way home from school powered by three fish sticks (each the size of a stick of chewing gum) that I had allowed myself for lunch due to the fact that I had skipped breakfast that morning as a result of waking up late yet again.

The journey from school to home was about 3 miles down a dusty gravel road past the county hospital and miles from anything else. It was an unseasonably hot spring day in Iowa and as I made my way down the road for home carrying a full load of books in the blistering midday sun. It was a struggle that day just to put one foot in front of the other in my weakened state. Then it happened; a feeling of *total surrender* washed over me. My body had finally "hit the wall". There was nothing left to give.

As my knees buckled and my eyes rolled back up into my head and the last thing I remember seeing was the pale blue sky above me immediately followed by the sight of the gravel road rushing at me as I slammed *face first* into the gravel road below… *"Ouch!…"*

"Hey kid, are you all right?"

I awoke to the site of the middle-aged man leaning over me franticly attempting to pry my eyelids open to dilate my pupils with a flashlight. He was an ambulance driver returning to the hospital after an out-of-town run. He had discovered me collapsed alongside the road, scooped me up and delivered me to the nearby hospital. Later I would learn that I had suffered a mild cardiac "episode" and they had administered CPR to revive me.

After hearing the news, I laid there on the E.R. table with the taste of gravel dust still in my mouth feeling a whole range of emotions- Shame, desperation, embarrassment, anger! What was I going to tell my mom? What will the kids at school say when they hear about this? Surely everybody will think it was drugs! Sure, it's always drugs… But I knew better. The truth was I almost died that day because I was so desperate for change that I was willing to do whatever it took no matter how radical... no matter how foolish… or how dangerous.

Round two

Fast-forward to my college years, I managed to hold together a reasonable diet that kept me at a fairly respectable weight – chalk that up to active 20-year-old metabolism and lack of access to moms' cooking, it wasn't like I was doing anything on purpose…

As I progressed from my 20s into my 30s and then into my 40s I developed a condition that causes calcium deposits to form in my joints making it impossible to straighten or bend my elbows or my knees unless I'm constantly moving. This makes any form of active exercise nearly impossible. And as a result of my limited activity the weight was starting to come back year-by-year to 260, 270, 290… And then the unthinkable, **305 pounds!**

"305 pounds…. Jesus!" I thought to myself "I weigh more than the other three members of my family all put

together! That's absolutely unacceptable!"
Okay, well I've identified the problem so what the hell am I going to do about it?

Clearly my history with weight loss to this point had not been impeccable to say the least and at 46 years old I knew my body would never handle the abuse that I gave it the first time around. This time I was going to have to be smarter about it.

As luck would have it I caught a program called ***Fat, sick and nearly dead***. It's the story of an overweight Aussie exec who visited America and decided to put himself on a *juice fast* as he crossed the country speaking with people about their thoughts on the typical American diet. Day by day he would document his results and as the film progresses you could literally see the pounds coming off.

I was intrigued. I watch the show several times and was impressed by the results but I was disappointed by the fact that despite making the movie and showing some impressive weight loss, there was not really much information given about the exact diet he was using, the schedule he was keeping to and/or exercise he was implementing (if any) to get his results.

Armed with what little information I could glean from the film and my own independent research, I initially set out to replicate his results ***the result of this book is a day by day account (for better or worse) of exactly what I did and how I did it.*** I don't want to paint a picture of an easy program and make you think that it's not hard because, it *is* hard. But I can tell you this: it does get easier after the first week and every day after that it gets even easier.

Since undertaking the first 30 days of my initial weight loss I have spoken with many professionals and dietary experts who have commended me on my approach and the problem solving methodology I have applied to create this program. And I can truly say it's unlike anything you've probably ever seen or tried before – *and best of all, it works - every single time!*

It's my honest wish for you as a reader to benefit from the effort I put into developing this program. If I can save just one life beyond my own I will consider my work a success.

Here's to you and YOUR transformation!

How To Kill A Diet In 3 Easy Steps

The first few days of the program are the hardest for most folks. To get through this initial period it is essential that you use every mental and physical trick in the bag to keep your focus on your goal and achieve your goals.

Within a few days though something magical begins to happen – *it gets easier. Things began to normalize and a familiar routine sets in. this is when you know "you've got it".*

Here's a few things that helped me quite a bit get through the hard times. Take these observations seriously because if you do you'll notice things go a lot more smoothly for you.

Diet Killer #1: Underestimating the urge to chew

This is a powerful drive that seems to be hardwired right into our DNA. After all, it's a survival instinct. It's remarkable how powerful this urge really is. If you were to go a couple of days on a straight liquid diet, you would literally begin to get an overwhelming feeling of *depression* (Which in turn would kick in your need to eat to alleviate bad feelings) - the feeling is as if some intangible thing is missing from your life, *that's because it is!*

Because it would be unrealistic for the first time in your life to think that you could just stop doing it *cold turkey* we need a way to satisfy this urge without undermining our plan. The biggest problem with having the urge to chew is we have to have something to *chew on*. This typically leads to munching and munching leads to falling off the program!

Luckily we can solve our need to chew without adding calories by carrying sugar free gum. When you begin to get the "munchies" 9 times out of 10 it's not *true hunger* it's just your body wanting to satisfy its need to chew. The solution? Pop a stick or two of gum in your mouth and watch how quickly the thought of snacking subsides.

Diet Killer #2: Running familiar patterns

Another reason we eat when were not really hungry is because the activity goes hand-in-hand with something we familiarize the act of eating with such as sitting in front of the TV, or going out to a movie.

Our brains, while remarkable, still operate in a primitive "*if-then*" form of basic programming installed in us by years of input from advertising, social programming, early parental influence and more.

For example: "*If* I go to a movie-*then* that means I need popcorn!"

Well, of course you don't *need* the popcorn. That's ridiculous. But, through repetition and failing to actively interrupt this pattern, over time you may have programmed yourself quite *automatically* to reach for that large tub of buttered popcorn when you're taking in the latest Hollywood blockbuster whether you really want it or not!

These *patterns* play out in many different ways hour upon hour all throughout our daily lives. And it's your job to actively recognize them for what they are.

Patterns are not legitimate hunger signals they are something *entirely different.*

Your focus throughout the next 30 days will be to recognize these patterns and interrupt them before they get started. To do so requires being able to recognize the *trigger*.

Triggers come in many forms. They can be a sight, a sound, or situation. They may even be a person.

For example:
Those of you of a certain age will remember the good humor ice cream man. At one point in time in America legions of these ice cream vendors slowly drove trucks around the streets of America accompanied by a loudspeaker on top playing the familiar good humor tune*. This tune became a trigger in the minds of a generation of children to the point that much like Pavlov's famous dogs, children began to salivate at the sound of the ice cream trucks siren song and they would come running in droves!

Your success for the next 30 days will be dependent upon your ability to recognize the triggers in your daily life and even to proactively avoid them as much as possible.

*Interestingly enough, the stronger the trigger the more durable and long lasting the effect. I wonder how many adults that grew up with the good humor man would still respond to that music even today!

Diet Killer #3: Inconsistent Intake

One of the *classics of diet failure* is the infamous *feast* and *famine* technique.
It goes something like this: A person will over eat and

to compensate for it will double down on their dieting and restrict their eating for the next day or two to make up. And it never works because you're pushing of the body's natural *"panic button."*

Your body has powerful protective measures in place to carry you through the *hard times* of no food. These days we don't have such things as "hard times" as compared with our primitive ancestors. But our bodies still operate exactly the same way as they always have.

No doubt you're aware that when you starve yourself your body goes into *power down* mode during this time it does its best to forcefully preserve what it deems to be the last of its reserves for an unforeseen time. Conversely, any massive uptake of food beyond what it deems to be immediately necessary dumps into its backup storage cells (fat) for later use.

It really is a simple system, but the diet industry has you thinking there some bigger mystery to what is *really* going on.

Once you understand what's going on, then correcting the mistakes you're making couldn't be any simpler. **Here's literally everything you need to know to lose weight:**

- Never go longer than four hours without eating *something.*
- Never take in more calories than you burn off on a day-to-day basis
- Be sure to consistently drink water all throughout the day

- Limit your intake of processed, animal-based or unnatural man made foods (that also includes dairy, cheese and bread and oh yes, diet soda!)

That's it! That's all you need to know… Seriously. If you follow these four rules you will lose weight – GUARANTEED.

I refer to these guidelines as the *4 pillars of success* and we will be taking a more detailed look at each of them in the next chapter.

The 4 Pillars Of Success

#1 Never go longer than four hours without eating something.

The conventional thinking is breakfast is the *most* important meal of the day. That's totally incorrect! *Every meal is important.* In fact you need more than just 3.

By keeping food in your system every four hours. You are allowing your digestion to work full cycle (provided you are in taking natural foods which take less time to process in your system then things like red meat and processed foods) and at the same time resetting your bodies *"preservation switch"* that flips on when you go into *starvation mode* – which starts surprisingly as soon as six hours after your last meal!

By consistently sending your body the message *"Everything is fine – there is no shortage of food"* it will not be compelled to slow down your metabolism to preserve its stores, nor will you even experience a lack of energy, a slowdown in brain function or any of the things associated with the onset of *starvation mode* symptoms.

To be clear here when I say *"eat every four hours"* what I'm talking about is taking in just a *bare minimum* of food, such as a handful of grapes or a glass of natural green veggie juice (I call it "Mean Green"). I'll go into more detail about that in my next point but your objective should be about every four waking hours to take in something that contains *some* amount of calories so that your body recognizes it as food. (Water and diet cola does not qualify).

Even the most stringent dieter will struggle from time to time to be successful at weight loss once hunger becomes a part of the picture. Our bodies produce a hormone known as **_ghrelin_**, which regulates hunger and in turn drives our appetite. Failure to understand, monitor and keep control of our ghrelin hormone level is what leads to failure. Cutting edge research tells us the best way to control this all-powerful hormone is to eat small, equally distributed meals (chronologically and calorically speaking) every 3 to 4 hours.

Timing is the key to everything!
By now you're probably wondering "what's so special about eating every 3 to 4 hours?" Research has demonstrated that ghrelin will spike after about 3 to 4 hours of fasting, therefore eating with well-timed regularity prevents _tripping the hunger trigger_. It should also be noted that ghrelin will spike if we deprive ourselves of carbs as well. So it is vitally important to make sure a portion of what we're putting our system provides those necessary carbs components to supply our bodies and brains the fuel they need.

When we take lazy "diet shortcuts" by skipping meals we are only inviting ghrelin spikes which will increase our hunger and cause cravings for sugar as well as affect us emotionally and energetically and thereby set up a scenario in which we will absolutely fail sooner or later.

#2 Never take in more calories than you burn off on a day-to-day basis

By now I think we're all pretty familiar with this concept, but few of us know *how to correctly apply* it.

In the last section we discussed the hormone ghrelin and how to regulate it via *consistent caloric intake throughout the day* but we haven't specified what that is… until now.

A man of *average size* seeking to lose weight safely, on a daily basis, should take in no more than 2000 calories and no less than 1200. An average sized woman should do no more than 1800 or less than 1000.* (For clarity here when I say *"size"* I mean *height not your current weight*.)

Using the above guidelines a typical male following **the 30 day burn program** consuming a 2000 calorie diet would be consuming an average of 400 calories about every four waking hours. The actual daily schedule timeline would look something like this:

7 AM Breakfast burrito: Corn tortilla filled with two scrambled eggs, sautéed onions, 1/4 cup of black beans and pico de gallo. This meal *Contains 30 grams of protein*. And serves as a hunger deterrent throughout the day.

11 AM Mean green smoothie – A big part of **The 30 Day Burn (T30DB)** program.

3 PM 2 Granola Bars *(My personal favorite is chocolate chip, peanut butter & pretzel!)*

5:30 PM Mean green smoothie #2 (or one of the others listed at back of this book.)

9:30 PM Mean green smoothie #3 – This serves 2 purposes: First, to aid in detoxifying your system from all those years of abuse and fat buildup and second, to flush out solid food in your system before you sleep.

Don't feel like you have to be a *stickler about exact times or the food example above.*
I've literally ate Oreo cookies for breakfast and still kept things on track!

If you want to see something really outrageous -
Check out my diet blog: TheOreoCookieDiet. at

http://theoreocookiedietblog.wordpress.com

*WHAT YOU EAT DOESN'T REALLY MATTER AS LONG AS THE TOTAL INTAKE OF CALORIES FOR EACH 4 HOUR CYCLE ARE CORRECT.

As you begin to understand how the system works, you'll soon realize **there really are no restrictions on what you can have The only rule is you absolutely must maintain the caloric guidelines of no more than 400 calories per meal (or 350 calories for you gals) Believe it or not, a slice of pizza, a small hamburger at McDonald's, even Ice cream or chocolate and cake as your snack are acceptable!*

The key thing to keep in mind here is you want to be eating no sooner than 3 and no later than 5 hours between meals and you're averaging every meals intake at your given **4 hour caloric allowance**.

*2000 calories / over 5 meals for the day yields a 400 calorie allowance per meal.

*These are general figures and apply to a fairly large part of the population however, if you're larger than average or smaller than average you should adjust

your figure up or down by about 100 calories to compensate.

*Ladies: you should adjust your TOTAL INTAKE to around 1750 to 1800 a day –
That works out to about 350 calories per sitting.*

#3 Be sure to consistently drink water all throughout the day

This rule is such an important one it should probably be first. It's been demonstrated that you can last a few weeks without food but only a matter of days without water. Water is so critical to the function of every part of your body that without it the whole system breaks down rather quickly.

For the purposes of losing weight, water serves another very critical role as well; it serves as the *primary transport system* to expel used material, (such as toxins and old fat known as lipids) from the body*.

You want to have *every opportunity possible* to get that fat out of your body *as fast as possible* and you don't want to create a *traffic jam* in your system by reducing the opportunities to expel waste due to a lack of water intake.

How much is too much or too little?
I'm not suggesting you drown yourself by constantly chugging water to the point where you slosh when you walk and I have a bit of a personal problem when experts tell us that we need to drink 8 - 8 oz. glasses a day! That's insanely time consuming and unsustainable as a lifestyle for most people.

The truth is most of the foods you already eat are water based and therefore are adding to your total liquid intake by virtue of their makeup. As for the rest of it?

Do what feels right. Personally I try to work in 2 to 3 big 32oz glasses a day if it works with my schedule.

Here's a fun fact: I can always tell when I'm in fat burning mode when I pee by the amount of foam I create! Foamy pee is created by high lipid content that happens to make your pee bubbly. Childish? Sure, but it still makes the little kid in me giggle. Girls, I'm sorry but this is a guy thing, you'll just have to take my word for it. Lol.

#4 Limit your intake of processed, animal-based or unnatural foods

For the next 30 days you will be on primarily what could be described as a plant-based diet. So this pillar will naturally take care of itself. However once you have finished *the 30 day burn program* you will need to strictly monitor your adherence to this one most of all.

Studies have routinely shown that diets high in animal-based and processed type foods (as I stated before this includes dairy, cheese and bread) are the biggest culprits when it comes to weight gain, sickness and disease as well as leading providers of "empty calories."

Don't shoot the messenger! I'm not suggesting that you completely cut out all your favorite foods for the rest of your life. I'm simply saying you need to consider how they fit in to your new lifestyle and in what portions and how often. Personally I still enjoy a small serving of steak on Friday night. I can't imagine life without it.

The Weigh in

Famed financial guru Peter Drucker once said *"what gets measured gets improved."* I couldn't agree more. That thinking applies to more than just money though, it applies to that spare tire around your midsection as well!

Part of the reason people get disillusioned with most diets is that they don't take an accurate look at where they are starting from and they couple that with unrealistic daily progress expectations. Fortunately for you this program takes that into account. You'll be able to measure your day-to-day progress against realistic expectations and know when you're falling behind and when you're exceeding your goals.

Before you begin

In order to track your progress **you're going to need a scale**. I highly suggest a digital scale so that you can track your losses down to a 1/10th of a pound (*I bought mine at bed Bath and beyond for about 60 bucks*). Most scales in this price range and above also display body fat percentage readouts as well as other information that can be usable too but it's not required for this program.

You're going to need a juicer (not a blender). Juicers operate by separating the pulp from the juice by spinning the whole thing at high speed without mixing it all together. If money is tight you could cheat and use a blender then strain the contents before drinking. Do what works and just don't get hung up on the mechanical issues.

Next **you are going to need a notebook** to do your daily journal entries. Don't overlook the importance of this simple tool because it really is a tremendous morale booster for you when times get hard and you feel your willpower slipping. It also helps to be able to look back at the last week's progress and reassure yourself that your efforts are paying off.

Those of you who prefer a more high tech approach to journaling might want to do a daily blog or online journal. For that I suggest *Blogger.com* (best of all it's free) the point here is to document your daily progress in some way. .

I encourage you to follow my advice and give yourself an honest daily account of your progress. It's remarkably therapeutic and serves as a motivating reminder later on of how far you've come and how much you overcame).

Consistency is critical

One of the keys to getting good results is consistent measurement at the same time every day, under the same circumstances and even using the same scale. You might be surprised to see how wildly your weight fluctuates throughout an average day (as much as 3 to 4 pounds or more!). To address this problem we pick *one set time each day – MORNING IS BEST* - to log our results and then stay off the scale for the rest of the day…(*Seriously, I mean it! Stay off the damn scale!* Watching your weight fluctuate up and down several times a day will just mess with your head and create a false sense of progress …or more likely a lack thereof).

Should you do "before and after" Pictures?

Yes! Nothing will motivate you to keep up the good work more than looking back at pictures of yourself on day one and seeing how rapidly your body has changed. You're going to be shocked by what you see.

I consider this a private motivator and not one that I share with anyone and you may consider it the same thing. So it goes without saying that stripping down to your underwear to take pictures is the best way to do it. Get your digital camera, go in to the bathroom and take a few pictures of yourself in the mirror. One from the front, one from the side and one from the back. Now hide them away and be prepared to be absolutely amazed in 7 days!

Ready? – Set? – Go!

I have found that the best time to check my progress is during my morning routine (7am). I wake up, empty my bladder and/or bowels and step on the scale to chart my progress for the day, jot down my thoughts about the preceding day's events and my feelings about them.

Once you have decided what time of day will be best for you to track your progress, and you have recorded your starting weight it's time to go shopping for supplies.

Day 1 Jumping In

Before getting started you need to know where you are currently in order to tell when you are making improvements. So let's do that now.

Beginning first thing in the morning with your bowels and bladder empty, strip off your clothes and step on your new digital scale to take your *starting point reading* and record it in your journal *(You did get a journal or set one up online right, right?)* If you spent the extra bucks to get one of the fancier scales that gives you a percentage of body fat readout among other things it doesn't hurt to record that information alongside the basics too (although it's not critical to this program).

Now that we have a reference point for your starting weight we can begin putting together the daily regimen of your **7 day test drive of the30dayburn** plan.

Below you will find the components used to make the basic *MEAN GREEN COCKTAIL* which is the starting point for the 30 day burn program. The recipe consists of one serving, tripling that amount will produce enough for one full day's use and is suggested to save you time and cleanup effort.

Always be sure to keep leftover amounts refrigerated and never produce more than one days use at a time to prevent *cellular breakdown* in the various components. It's also a good idea to never let your juices sit longer than 12 hours before consuming them.

Critical note: Morning weigh-ins should always be done after you have emptied your bladder (and preferably your bowels as well) for the most consistent tracking results. You are always at your lightest first thing in the morning before you begin to take in liquids and eat so I find taking readings at this time of day to be far more consistent to any other based upon this fact alone.

Diet components

Because this is only a 7 day test drive, and we won't have much opportunity to vary your diet day by day, each of your days eating schedules generally all breakdown like this:

A couple of scrambled eggs in the morning with juice
Followed by your first smoothie around 11 AM.
At about 3 PM you'll have a couple of granola bars
And another smoothie and about 5 to 5:30 PM with your evening dinner.
Your last smoothie comes about 9 to 9:30.
Intake of water throughout the day is recommended to assist in flushing out your system.

A closer look at the essential components
Eggs - Early on in my research I got hip to the side benefits of eggs as a source of dietary support. They are generally low in fat and very high in protein and that makes for an excellent jumpstart for your day. The protein component serves a double purpose as well. Recent research has demonstrated that protein, taken in moderate amounts in the morning, acts as an appetite suppressant with effects reaching all the way into the middle of the day. With great news like that, *why wouldn't* you want to start your day with eggs?

The Mean green cocktail – this is the staple of the entire program. It provides what I euphemistically refer to as the *trash collection* component of the diet. Because every component within the cocktail is comprised of *green* fruits and vegetables they are very high in essential nutrients and alkalinity.

The modern Western diet is filled with so much acidity it's absolutely horrifying! This acidity backs up in your system year after year, leading to a whole host of ailments, of which obesity is but one.

By flushing your system out twice a day with an *alkaline wash*, you're giving your body a chance to *reboot* its built-in defenses and do what it already has a natural ability to do under optimum circumstances- In our case that would be drop the unwanted weight!

HOW TO MAKE The MEAN GREEN COCKTAIL:
- 1 or 2 large green apples
- 1 Large pack of celery
- 1 Lemon or lime (don't use the outer rind)
- 1 Big cluster of broccoli head and stalk
- 2 large cucumbers
- Wheatgrass powder – (I get mine online)

Prepare your juice and drink right away or prepare the above recipe X3 for full days use and refrigerate (Note: Juice should never be stored longer than 12 hours due to cellular breakdown)

Granola bars – I chose to add granola bars as part of the basic diet regimen for many reasons, mainly because I wanted to have something with some *"bulk"* to it, as I realized a strictly liquid diet would leave me feeling empty all the time. Traditional granola contains oats, which expand in the stomach and allow you to feel fuller, faster- and it does so with a minimum number of calories taken in.

Besides adding a second dose of protein to your diet, granola produces a natural internal *"scrubbing effect"*, helping to knock loose all the junk that's built up in your digestive tract.

The right kind of granola bars don't have to cost you a fortune either. I've discovered some of the best granola bars I've ever had in my life under a store generic brand name. If you happen to be fortunate enough to live in the Midwest of America, try *Hy-Vee stores private label granola bars. Their peanut butter, chocolate pretzel granola bars* are insanely good, and only two bucks for a box of eight!

Want more options?
**Check out the sugar free snack cookbook
by Betty Jean**

http://bit.do/sugarfree

There is no need to go crazy buying expensive brand-name granola bars, and I do not suggest you opt for the expensive protein bars that are so common these days. You're mainly looking for product with around 100 calories per serving. It doesn't matter if you like peanut butter, chocolate chip white chocolate or traditional fruit and nut type granolas. They all work the same as long as you keep to my hundred calorie recommendation.

The Great Diet Plan Deception

By now you've come to realize that losing weight really isn't really all that difficult.
So why has it taken so long to this point to produce the results you've always wanted?
The answer is very simple: ***marketing!***

If it were not for special *buzzwords*, patented routines, printed additional materials or a particular focus on a few key ingredients, there would be nothing separating one diet fad from the next. Therein lies the grand deception.

The first rule of magic is to never let the viewer see what the other hand is doing.
This is sort of the way the diet industry works, they would have you believe that it is their *patented one-of-a-kind special diet system **and not the calorie count*** that is responsible for your weight loss. As you are starting to see, nothing could be further from the truth!

Falling Off The Plan

"To error is human"
- Alexander Pope from an essay on criticism

It happens to the best of us, a moment of weakness or a failing to make good on our plans, to recognize this is to understand that we are all fallible and prone to temptation.

In full disclosure I too had been tempted by the siren song of a Snickers bar during this program and have succumbed to moment of weakness. That's no reason to beat yourself up though. Remember; this is a *lifestyle*, not a race. There is no finish line. Learning to eat properly is a skill that must be practiced and built up over time.

I have found it helpful after a moment of weakness to adopt the attitude that *the next thing I eat will be the right thing*. There's no sense in waiting until tomorrow or next week to restart the program. Simply recognize your mistake and continue on with the next meal as if no great sin has occurred. This will prevent you from creating excuses or losing any momentum.

In the next chapter you'll get a preview of how to turn a potential moment of weakness into a beneficial act.

Exercise Vs Stretching

By now you're probably wondering "When is he going to tell me to start exercising?" The answer is – *I'm not*. T30DB does not require the use of exercise to work. In fact, it can actually be counterproductive to the process of losing weight on this plan.

Now, don't get me wrong, I'm not down on exercise. By now you've discovered stores of energy you probably didn't even know you were capable of and you're probably chomping at the bit to burn some of it off. There's nothing wrong with that. A walk around the block or even a low impact bike ride is perfectly fine.

All I'm saying here is resist the urge (for now) to get involved in high impact cardio activities or weightlifting as they will send mixed signals to your body and can actually have the reverse effect or cause unintended setbacks.

Although it's not necessary to the program I do recommend stretching. While it's beyond the scope of this book to outline a stretching exercise routine there is an unlimited supply easily accessible online by searching Google any time you like.

By stretching you are enabling your body to *ring out* toxins from your muscle tissue much in the way that you would squeeze out water from a twisted towel. It takes just minutes a day, it's very low impact and it really works!

Just remember to keep plenty of water in your system because all that bad stuff has to have somewhere to go and it needs some way to exit your body.

How To Eat Anything You Want

I'm about to ruin everything you *think* you know about diets.
If I were to tell you that you could eat a dozen donuts for breakfast, an entire bag of chocolate chip cookies, as a midday snack followed by unbridled portions of pizza for lunch and a full course meal at your favorite fast food restaurant (and you can even go ahead and supersize it)

Then if I were to tell you with a completely straight face that *this will help you lose weight*, would you think I was out of my friggin mind?
Yes, I'm sure you would… But that's exactly what I'm about to do.

While creating the initial T30DB program I stumbled upon some research that suggested that spiking caloric intake every 7 to 10 days can have a profound effect on long-term weight loss. I put this information on the back burner and did not include it in the original program however I want to make you aware that I have incorporated this into my continuing weight loss program (see chapter entitled the next 30 days in the full course version of this book) and have had outstanding results.

The science of splurging explained
It seems highly improbable doesn't it? After all, T30DB is based on the simple *calorie in – calorie out* model right? Yes, but nothing of life is ever *that simple*. There are always exceptions to the rule Let me explain. The latest research suggests *dietary plateaus* occur due to the body's constant need to regulate itself and set

baseline expectancies

Think of your body as a food warehouse. Your internal warehouse manager checks his deliveries each day and makes operational predictions based on available space for incoming and outgoing product. For example: if business is slow and product isn't coming in at a normally expected pace it makes no sense to keep the lights on in the entire building so certain sections of the building are shut down to be more efficient. Likewise, if business is booming employees may have to work double shifts to keep product moving in the given available space if not additional space will be needed and an expansion may be called for!

Continuing this far-fetched analogy let's assume our warehouse manager knows that one day a week an unusually heavy amount of product will flow through the warehouse. It's not worth expanding, and it's just not worth shutting down parts of the building. It simply keeps the employees on their toes knowing that there is a certain level of expectancy to be maintained to keep things running in good working order.

Therefore, taking this into account I instituted a *"seventh day of sin"* into the weekly diet regimen. Very simply put this allows for an unregulated intake of any and every food you desire! I shoot for Sunday as it tends to be a very sedentary day and one where family and food go hand-in-hand.

Why does this work?
Scientific research into this subject indicates that when the body is faced with an extreme food situation (either too much or too little) it sees this situation as a need to adjust *baseline settings* such as metabolism, energy

consumption and fat storage. By "shocking" the system every 7 to 10 days you are keeping things in a state of "heightened awareness" – bodybuilders have known the same thing about muscle growth for years. If you do the same thing day after day the body will adapt and fail to respond. This is known as a plateau. The only way to break out is to do something out of the ordinary and totally unexpected. In other words...*OVER EAT!*

Won't that wipe out all my hard work?
No. remember the old comedy routine from the TV show I love Lucy where the gals take a job working in a candy factory? Their job is simple: as the candy comes down the conveyer belt it's their job to wrap each piece and pack it away and all goes well for a while.... Until they speed things up! Soon the girls are overwhelmed with candy flying at them faster and faster (much of it isn't even caught) and they are struggling just to pack it all away. (Sorry if I just exposed your age! You younger kids will have to check it out on Youtube for a good laugh) Your body will react the exact same way...IF, AND ONLY IF you do it once every 7 to 10 days and maintain the program I've outlined on every other day

Your body will think *"What the hell just happened? I better crank up the metabolism to make damn sure we're ready if this ever happens again!"*... Days go by, nothing happens (the expected massive food intake never comes) and your metabolism settles down and resets itself ...and then it's SHOCK TIME again!

If this all seems incredibly insane to you (or at best highly irresponsible) then you should know that these findings are backed up by the latest peer reviewed science.

Why hasn't this made big news? Just think about it…
If you were a diet pill maker would you want anyone to
think that EATING is actually a good thing?

The fact of the matter is that this method HAS been
highly researched and has been featured at
The30DayBurn.**Com** as well as other books such as
the 4 hour body by Tim Ferriss.

Both Tim and I go into a much greater bit of detail in
our larger books than I have space for in this small
report so If you're up for a good excuse to binge I
suggest you pick up a copy of both books.

I do want to be clear that overeating is a *technique* to
overcome hitting a level in your diet you simply can't
break through any other way. *It's not a lifestyle* and it is
NOT needed to succeed with the basics of my program.

For more information on the *Shock system* see the
complete program at www.The30DayBurn.Com

Sleep

Want to lose up to an incredible 3 pounds in less than 24 hours? Make a point of getting to bed earlier. Researchers from the University of Pennsylvania found that just a few nights of sleep deprivation can lead to an almost immediate weight gain.

Researchers asked participants in a sleep study to at least 10 hours of sleep a night for two days and then followed it up with five nights of restricted sleep and four more nights of recovery. After the 11 day study the sleep deprived group had gained almost 3 pounds compared to the control group putting in 10 hours a night.

The results of this study really shouldn't surprise anyone. When you think about it the main function of sleep is to shift the body's processes from *performance* to *maintenance*. This cycle is critical to proper function. Would you race a car nonstop for 24 hours without ever making a pit stop?

Sleep and fat loss-the hormone connection
Fat can wreak total havoc on your hormones and impair your ability to lose fat. For instance, hormones such as melatonin, serotonin, and dopamine influence motivation, mood, sleep, and hunger cravings. The correct natural growth hormone balance is essential because it handles growth and repair of your body. A deficiency in your hormonal balance promotes fat gain.

Sleep plays a critical role in regulating each of these hormones. It's time for a "sleep overhaul" if you find yourself regularly Googling: *"How can I get to sleep."*

The following list highlights some of the more common sleep-disrupting habits that can sabotage your slumber.

Sleep Mistake #1: Eating too close to bedtime.
Late-night meals and trips to the fridge prevent your body from slowing down during sleep as well as raising your insulin level. As a result, less cell-boosting melatonin and growth hormone are released into your system while you slumber

The cure:
Cut out all food and drink intake 3 yours or more before bed.

Sleep Mistake #2: Sleeping with too much light exposure or napping too close to your digital alarm clock.
Even just a small amount of light can disrupt the release of *melatonin* and, subsequently, the release of growth hormones. Research has also shown *cortisol* to remain abnormally high when sleeping subjects are exposed to light as well.

You should also be far away from *electromagnetic fields (EMFs)* emitted from electrical devices such as digital alarm clocks in your bedroom. These can disrupt the pineal gland and the production of melatonin and serotonin. (On a side note: research has also linked EMFs to increased risk of cancer so better to play it safe than be sorry for more than one reason.)

The Cure: Keep your sleeping area dark. The darker the better and keep electrical equipment at least 6 feet away, if you must use these items. It's best to turn the light display away from your line of sight.

Sleep Mistake #3: Drinking too much liquid before bed.

This can be an obvious one but we've all made the mistake many times. Drinking before bedtime can increase your need for late-night trips to the toilet. Waking up to pee interrupts your natural sleep rhythm and puts your whole body out of whack. If you turn the light on when you go, you also run the risk of suppressing melatonin production making things even more disruptive.

The Cure: Stop drinking three hours before bedtime and use a red night light in the bathroom, if a night light is needed at all (it really works!)

Sleep Mistake #4: Exercising late at night.

During the T30DB program you will not be required to exercise so this shouldn't be a problem while on this program but generally speaking for the rest of the population this one is a huge *"no-no"* for sleep deprived among us.

There is little doubt exercise can certainly help you sleep better, so long as you do it at the proper time (I suggest mid-morning). A late-night workout, especially cardio, substantially raises core body temperature, preventing the release of melatonin. It can also interfere with your ability to relax and drift off to sleep, since it usually spikes noradrenaline, dopamine, and cortisol, which stimulate brain activity, which is not a recipe for a good night sleep (who among us hasn't had the experience of a sleepless night due to mind that won't calm down and stop buzzing away?)

The Cure: Avoid any form of cardiovascular exercise in the final 3-hour period before bed.

Sleep Mistake #5: Too much TV or computer use before bed.

Many folks enjoy watching their favourite TV shows, catching up on emails, or just surfing the net in the evenings, but too much time in front of either screen close to bedtime has also been shown to interfere with a good night's sleep. These activities increase the stimulating hormones noradrenaline and dopamine, which as you now know hamper your ability to fall asleep.

The Cure: Set aside 30 minutes prior to sleep to "power down" and focus on mind-calming activities such as meditation or reading a book (*Not a lighted screen type e-reader or kindle!*) These habits will surely boost serotonin and improve your sleep.

Sleep Mistake #6: Keeping your bedroom too warm.

I know it feels cozy at bedtime, but a bedroom that's too

warm can prevent an essential *natural cool down* that should take place in your body as you sleep.

Without this cooling process, melatonin and growth-hormone release is disrupted, that means you won't be burning fat while you sleep or benefiting from night-time repair your bones, skin, and muscles require.

The Cure: Try to sleep in a cool area, ideally below 70 degrees Fahrenheit.

Sleep Mistake #7: Sleeping in tight-fitting clothes.
It's true, your favorite PJs really can actually help you sleep better, but not if they're too tight. It's been shown that tightly fitting clothing at bedtime--even a bra or underwear-- raises your body temperature and this too has been proven to reduce secretion of melatonin and growth hormone.

The Cure: Sleep in the nude and avoid excessive, heavy blankets. If you prefer to wear something to bed, make sure it's light weight, made from breathable fabric and is above all else loose fitting.

Sleep Mistake #8: Failure to open the blinds or go outside in the morning.
Remember, melatonin is supposed to be lowest first thing in the morning. If you stay in darkness, your body will not pick up the signal that the time has come to get up and go.

High melatonin levels during the day leaves you feeling groggy, fatigued and unable to fully wake up properly. It may also possibly lower serotonin, this leads to depression, anxiety, and those wicked, diet killing hunger cravings.

The Cure: Crack open the curtains and throw open the shutters! Let the light in as soon as you open your eyes. Send a clear signal to yourself that the day has begun!

Sleep Mistake #9: Not getting the right amount of sleep.
New research recently reported that people who regularly sleep 7½ hours per night live longer. The American Cancer Association found higher incidences of cancer in individuals who consistently slept six hours or less or more than nine hours nightly.

Most sleep experts agree that seven to eight hours a night is optimal. However, some people may require more or less sleep than others. If you wake without an alarm in the morning and feel refreshed when you get up, you're likely getting the right amount of sleep for you.

When your sleep is insufficient, your cortisol and hunger hormones both surge, causing a corresponding increase in insulin. You also experience decreases in leptin, melatonin, growth hormone, testosterone, and serotonin, all of which lead to weight gain.

The Cure: Aim for 7½ to nine hours nightly.

Sleep Mistake #10: Going to bed too late.
Staying awake until the wee hours causes hormonal imbalance because it increases cortisol, decreases leptin, and depletes growth hormone. It can also cause us to eat more, and it messes with our metabolism.

Cortisol naturally begins to increase during the second half of your sleep--a small boost at 2 a.m., another at 4 a.m., and the peak at around 6 a.m. If you're just getting to bed immediately beforehand, you're missing out on your most restful period of sleep.

More than half the respondents to the 2005 National Sleep Survey reported they are morning people with higher energy earlier in the day, while 41 percent considered themselves night owls. Evening people were more likely than morning people to experience symptoms of insomnia and sleep apnea, enjoy less sleep than they felt they needed, and take longer to fall asleep.

The Cure: Hit the sack between 10 and 11 p.m.

Going Deeper Into The Program

Congratulations! You've gotten your first taste of my program and I know *for a fact* that if you followed along you've gotten some pretty positive results. That being said, I'm sure you're anxious to keep those results going!

Now is the time to head on over to my website and grab a FULL COPY of the program. I have so much more to teach you and a few free gifts as well.

www.The30DayBurn.Com

Once again I'd like to thank you for your purchase and I'd like to ask you to take time to leave a positive review for others to finally find a little light in the diet darkness. Your success with this program means everything to me.

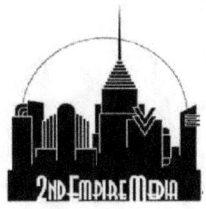

2ND EMPIRE MEDIA

Check out these other titles:

The Sugar Free Snack Cook Book
Featuring 80 Delicious Recipes.

http://bit.do/sugarfree

...

The Stubborn Fat Cure
Say Goodbye To Those
Hard To Lose Love Handles

http://bit.do/stubbornfat